EMBRACING A LIFE OF OPTIMAL WELLBEING

By

Olaitan Onakoya

ISBN: 9798870581217

First published, 2023

Published by:

Scentury Corporate Publishers Ltd.,

Suite 6, Jadesola Shopping Complex,

Olaogun Bus Stop, Old Ife Road, Ibadan, Oyo State, Nigeria.

Tel: +(234) 8033941355

E-mail: oyedeleolad@gmail.com

Table of Contents

Dedication 4

Acknowledgments 5

Introduction 6

CHAPTER ONE: Understanding Well-Being 9

CHAPTER TWO: Nurturing the Physical Body 13

CHAPTER THREE: Cultivating Mental Well-Being.....21

CHAPTER FOUR: Emotional Intelligence and Emotional Health 27

CHAPTER FIVE: Finding Purpose and Meaning.........35

CHAPTER SIX: Balancing Work and Life 42

CHAPTER SEVEN: Cultivating Positive Habits and Practices 48

CHAPTER EIGHT: Environmental Well-Being 54

CHAPTER NINE: Overcoming Challenges and Resilience...63

References...73

About the Book...74

About the Author..76

Dedication

This book is dedicated to Almighty God and to the memory of my loving and caring mother, Late Princess (Mrs.) Jokotola Adesola Onakoya.

Acknowledgments

I wish to express my deepest gratitude to my family – their unflinching believe in me, their patience during the countless hours, and their willingness to make sacrifices to accommodate my writing schedules have been the driving force behind the completion of this book. Without their unconditional love, constant encouragement and words of wisdom, this accomplishment would not have been possible.

I am indebted to my esteemed publisher and my brilliant editor, whose invaluable guidance, insightful feedback, and dedication to excellence have played a pivotal role in shaping this book into the refined work it has become. Their patience and understanding throughout the entire process have been truly remarkable.

Last but not least, I ascribe all glory, honour, and praise to Almighty God, the source of all wisdom and knowledge. It is through His divine grace and favour that I have been able to navigate the challenges of balancing my professional and personal commitments while still finding the time and inspiration to pen these words. This book is a testament to the boundless possibilities that can be achieved when one aligns with the divine plan.

Introduction

Welcome to the Journey Towards Achieving Optimal Well-Being

In this quest for a healthier and happier life, we'll explore various aspects of physical, mental, and emotional well-being. Together, we will discover practical tips, insights, and strategies to help you live a more balanced and fulfilling life. So, let's embark on this journey towards a brighter and healthier future.

Having worked in a health sector for some years, I always feel the pains that patients with disability go through.

I have related with many patients that have health challenges. I realised during our conversa-tion that some patients usually applied wrong treatment in solving their health challenges.

When their health status deteriorate, that is when they will have to start looking for medical help.

There are certain steps human being can take to preserve their health than seeking medical help all the time.

It is one of the reasons that prompted me to write Embracing A Life of Optimal Well-Being.

The Importance of Physical, Mental, and Emotional Well-Being

Physical, mental, and emotional well-being are integral components of a fulfilling and balanced life. Here's why they are so crucial:

Physical Well-Being: Your physical health forms the foundation of overall well-being. It impacts your energy levels, immune system, and longevity. By maintaining a healthy diet, regular exercise, and adequate sleep, you reduce the risk of chronic illnesses, boost your vitality, and enhance your quality of life.

Mental Well-Being: Mental health is equally vital. A sound mind is key to making clear decisions, managing stress, and achieving personal and professional goals. When your mental well-being is prioritised, you can enhance resilience, cope with life's challenges, and foster positive relationships.

Emotional Well-Being: Emotions play a significant role in daily life. Acknowledging and managing your emotions can lead to increased self-awareness and better relationships with others. Emotional well-being allows you to experience a range of emotions while also developing emotional intelligence and coping mechanisms.

Collectively, these dimensions of well-being impact each other. When they are in harmony, you are more likely to live a fulfilling and purpose-driven life. Conversely, neglecting one aspect can lead to imbalances, thereby negatively impacting one's overall quality of life. Therefore, striving for optimal physical, mental, and emotional well-being is a worthy and holistic pursuit.

Setting the Intention to Prioritise and Cultivate a Balanced and Fulfilling Life

To prioritise and cultivate a balanced and fulfilling life, start by setting clear goals, managing your time effectively, nurturing relationships, practising self-care, and pursuing your passions. Time is a resources which must be judiciously used. Nowadays, social media have taken people time. Some people do not build good relationship. Consistency and mindfulness will be key in achieving this balance.

CHAPTER ONE: Understanding Well-Being

Well-being refers to a person's overall state of health, happiness, and prosperity. It encompasses physical, mental, emotional, and social aspects of life. Factors contributing to well-being include good physical health, positive mental and emotional states, meaningful relationships, a sense of purpose, financial stability, and a supportive community. Achieving and maintaining well-being is a holistic endeavour that involves balance and attention to various life domains.

Defining Well-Being and Its Various Dimensions

Well-being is a broad concept that encompasses the overall quality of life and the state of an individual's physical, mental, and social health. It includes various dimensions:

Physical Well-Being: This dimension refers to the state of an individual's physical health. It involves factors such as nutrition, exercise, sleep, and access to healthcare.

Mental Well-Being: Mental well-being encompasses emotional and psychological health. It includes aspects like emotional stability, stress management, resilience, and a positive mindset.

Social Well-Being: Social well-being relates to the quality of an individual's social relationships and interactions. It involves factors such as social support, a sense of belonging, and the ability to maintain healthy relationships.

Economic Well-Being: Economic well-being is tied to an individual's financial situation and economic security. It includes factors like personal disposable income, employment, financial stability, and access to resources.

Environmental Well-Being: This dimension pertains to the relationship between an individual and their surroundings. It involves factors such as access to clean air and water, a safe and sustainable environment, and the ability to connect with nature.

Spiritual Well-Being: Spiritual well-being is often associated with a sense of purpose and meaning in life. It can encompass religious or philosophical beliefs, personal values, and a connection to something greater than oneself.

Cultural Well-Being: Cultural well-being is influenced by an individual's cultural identity and heritage. It involves factors such as cultural acceptance, cultural engagement, and the preservation of cultural traditions.

Intellectual Well-Being: Intellectual well-being focuses on cognitive development and lifelong learning. It includes factors like education, intellectual stimulation, and the pursuit of knowledge and skills.

Occupational Well-Being: Occupational well-being relates to one's satisfaction and fulfillment in their work or chosen occupation. It involves factors such as job satisfaction, work-life balance, and career development.

These dimensions are interconnected, and achieving well-being often requires a balance across all of them. Different individuals may prioritise these dimensions differently. Cultural and personal factors can also play a significant role in shaping one's perception of well-being.

Exploring the Interconnectedness of Physical, Mental, and Emotional Health

The interconnectedness of physical, mental, and emotional health is a crucial aspect of overall well-being. Physical health, which includes aspects like diet, exercise, and sleep, can significantly impact mental and emotional well-being. Conversely, mental and emotional health can influence physical health. Maintaining a balance between these aspects is essential for a healthy and fulfilling life.

The impact of well-being on overall quality of life and personal fulfilment

It is an important components of overall quality of life and well being.The impact contribute significantly to an individual's perception of their life's value and fulfilment. Impact of well-being is strongly linked to someone happiness and life satisfaction.

We always look at the rich people as the most happy people in the world. We forget that they have their own problems.

In life, it is internal satisfaction that matter most. A poor person may have a good impact of well-being and personal fulfilment in life than a rich people.

CHAPTER TWO: Nurturing the Physical Body

Nurturing the physical body involves taking care of your physical health through various practices such as:

Healthy Diet: Eat a balanced diet rich in fruits, vegetables, lean proteins, and whole grains. Avoid excessive processed foods, sugars, and unhealthy fats. Eat a balanced diet rich in brain-boosting nutrients like omega-3 fatty acids antioxidants and vitamins.

Regular Exercise: Incorporate physical activity into your daily routine. Aim for a mix of aerobic, strength, and flexibility exercises. Physical activity can enhance blood flow to the brain and improve cognitive functions. Incorporate regular physical activity into your routine, whether it is daily walks, workouts or sports you enjoy. You can employ a trainer to train you on how to stay fit and healthy in a gym centre.

Adequate Sleep: Ensure you get enough quality sleep to allow your body to rest and recover. I ensure I get enough quality sleep to allow my body to rest and recover. I make sure that my sleeping hours is completed. Quality sleep allows the body to repair and recover, promoting optimal physical health.

Hydration: Drink plenty of water to stay hydrated. Limit sugary drinks and excessive caffeine. I have a number of drinking bottles of water I drink daily. It has been of great help to my body system.

Stress Management: Practise stress-reduction techniques like meditation, deep breathing or yoga.

Regular Check-ups: Visit your healthcare provider for routine check-ups and screenings to catch potential health issues early. Your ability to detect early disease will go a long way to cure the disease.

Limit Alcohol and Avoid Smoking: Limit alcohol consumption, and avoid smoking or tobacco products.

Sun Protection: Use sunscreen to protect your skin from harmful UV rays. You can use sun glasses to protect your eyes from bright sunlight.

Proper Hygiene: Maintain good personal hygiene practices to prevent illness and infections.

Balance Work and Rest: Avoid overworking yourself and ensure you take breaks to rest and recharge. When you over-work yourself during your youthful years, not having adequate rest, it can results to illness and disease when you are old.

Remember that nurturing your physical body is a crucial part of overall well-being and can positively impact your mental and emotional health as well.

A healthy lifestyle, encompassing exercise, nutrition, and sleep, is crucial for overall well-being. Here's the significance of each component:

Exercise

Physical fitness: Regular exercise helps maintain a healthy weight, build muscle, and improve cardiovascular health.

Mental well-being: It releases endorphins, reducing stress and anxiety while enhancing mood and cognitive function.

Disease prevention: Exercise lowers the risk of chronic conditions like heart disease, diabetes, and certain cancers.

Longevity: It promotes a longer, healthier life by improving overall vitality and reducing the risk of premature death.

Nutrition

Energy and vitality: Proper nutrition provides the body with essential nutrients and energy for daily activities.

Weight management: A balanced diet helps maintain a healthy weight, reducing the risk of obesity-related health issues.

Disease prevention: Good nutrition can lower the risk of chronic diseases like hypertension, diabetes, and osteoporosis.

Immune system support: A well-rounded diet strengthens the immune system, enhancing the body's ability to fight off infections.

Sleep

Physical health: Quality sleep allows the body to repair and recover, promoting optimal physical health.

Mental health: It is crucial for cognitive function, memory consolidation, and emotional well-being.

Stress reduction: Sufficient sleep helps manage stress and improves overall resilience.

Hormone regulation: Sleep is essential for regulating hormones, including those that control appetite and stress responses.

In combination, these elements of a healthy lifestyle create a synergistic effect, enhancing physical and mental health while reducing the risk of various diseases. Prioritising exercise, nutrition, and sleep can lead to a higher quality of life and increased longevity.

Creating a Personalised Fitness Routine that Aligns With Individual Goals and Interests

To create a personal fitness routine involves several steps:

Define Goals: Determine specific fitness goals, such as weight loss, muscle gain, or improved endurance.

Assess Current Fitness: Evaluate your current fitness level to establish a baseline.

Choose Activities: Select exercises and activities you enjoy as this increases adherence.

Set Frequency: Determine how often you can realistically work out each week.

Plan Duration: Decide on the length of each workout session.

Design Workouts: Create a balanced routine that includes cardiovascular, strength, flexibility and core exercises.

Progression: Gradually increase intensity, duration, or weight as you get fitter.

Nutrition: Align your diet with your fitness goals.

Rest and Recovery: Incorporate rest days for muscle recovery.

Monitor Progress: Keep track of your progress to make necessary adjustments.

Understanding the Importance of a Balanced and Nourishing Diet

A balanced and nourishing diet is crucial for maintaining good health. It provides essential nutrients, vitamins and minerals that support bodily functions, energy levels, and overall well-being. It can help prevent chronic diseases, promote healthy growth and contribute to a longer, more active life. Proper nutrition also supports a strong immune system and mental clarity.

Strategies for improving Sleep Quality and Establishing a Consistent Routine

-       **Set a Consistent Schedule**: Go to bed and wake up at the same time every day, even on weekends. This helps regulate your body's internal clock.

-       **Create a Relaxing Bedtime Routine:** Wind down before bed with calming activities like reading, taking a warm bath, or practising relaxation exercises.

-       **Limit Exposure to Screens:** Avoid electronic devices with screens (phones, computers, TVs) at least an hour before bedtime. The blue light can interfere with your sleep-wake cycle.

-       **Mind Your Diet:** Avoid heavy meals, caffeine, and alcohol close to bedtime. These can disrupt sleep patterns.

-       **Make Your Sleep Environment Comfortable:** Ensure your bedroom is cool, dark, and quiet. Invest in a comfortable mattress and pillows.

-       **Get Regular Exercise:** Regular physical activity can promote better sleep, but avoid intense workouts too close to bedtime.

-       **Manage Stress**: Practise stress-reduction techniques like meditation, deep breathing, or yoga to relax your mind and body.

-       **Limit Naps:** If you need to nap, keep it short (20-30 minutes) and earlier in the day to avoid interfering with night-time sleep.

-       **Watch Your Liquid Intake:** Reduce your fluid intake in the evening to minimise night-time awakenings to use the bathroom.

-       **Limit Clock Watching**: Staring at the clock can increase anxiety about not sleeping. If you can't sleep, get out of bed and do something relaxing until you feel sleepy.

-       **Seek Professional Help:** If sleep problems persist, consult a healthcare professional or sleep specialist to rule out underlying issues like sleep disorders.

Note: It may take some time for these strategies to have a noticeable effect, so be patient and consistent in your efforts to improve sleep quality and establish a healthy sleep routine. In the long run, you will still derive maximum benefit from all these practices.

CHAPTER THREE: Cultivating Mental Well-Being

Recognising and Managing Stress and Anxiety

Identify Triggers: Recognise what causes your stress and anxiety: Is it work, relationships, or specific situations? Understanding the triggers is the first step.

Practise Mindfulness: Mindfulness techniques, such as deep breathing and meditation, can help you stay present and reduce anxiety.

Exercise Regularly: Physical activity releases endorphins, which can improve mood and reduce stress.

Maintain a Healthy Diet: Eating well-balanced meals and avoiding excessive caffeine or alcohol can help stabilise your mood.

Set Realistic Goals: Manage expectations and set achievable goals to reduce feelings of overwhelm.

Time Management: Organise your tasks and prioritise them to reduce stress from feeling overwhelmed.

Seek Support: Don't hesitate to talk to friends, family, or a therapist about your feelings. Some-times, just sharing your thoughts can alleviate anxiety.

Practise Relaxation Techniques: Techniques like progressive muscle relaxation or guided imagery can help reduce stress.

Limit Exposure to Stressors: When possible, avoid or minimize exposure to situations or people that consistently trigger stress.

Consider Professional Help: If stress and anxiety are significantly impacting your life, consult a mental health professional for guidance and potential treatment options.

Remember, managing stress and anxiety is an ongoing process. What works best can vary from person to person, so it may take some trial and error to find the most effective strategies for you.

- **Developing Healthy Coping Mechanisms and Resilience**

Mindfulness and Meditation: These practices can help you stay grounded and reduce stress.

Social Support: Connect with friends and loved ones for emotional support. Interacting with others can stimulete your brain and provide a mental break.

Positive Self-Talk: Challenge negative thoughts and cultivate a more optimistic outlook.

Problem-Solving Skills: Learn to tackle problems methodically.

Time Management: Organise your tasks to reduce stress and increase productivity.

Seeking Professional Help: Therapy or counselling can provide valuable guidance.

Self-Care: Prioritise self-care activities to recharge and maintain balance.

Remember, building resilience takes time and effort, but it is a valuable skill that can improve your overall mental and emotional well-being.

Practising Mindfulness and Meditation for Mental Well-Being

Start with the Basics: Begin with short, guided mindfulness or meditation sessions. There are many apps and online resources available to help you get started.

Consistency is Key: Regular practice is more beneficial than occasional sessions. Try to establish a daily routine, even if it's just a few minutes.

Find a Quiet Space: Choose a peaceful and quiet environment to minimise distractions during your practise.

Focus on Breath: Pay attention to your breath as it goes in and out. This simple focus can anchor your mind and calm your thoughts.

Non-Judgemental Awareness: Practise observing your thoughts without judgement. Let them come and go like clouds in the sky.

Body Scan: Perform a body scan to notice and release tension or discomfort in different parts of your body.

Guided Meditations: Use guided meditations or apps that provide structured sessions with instructions and themes.

Mindful Walking: You can practise mindfulness while walking by paying attention to each step and the sensations in your body.

Progressive Muscle Relaxation: Combine meditation with progressive muscle relaxation techniques to reduce physical tension.

Set Intentions: Start your practice with a clear intention; whether it is to reduce stress, increase focus, or improve overall well-being.

Be Patient: It is normal for your mind to wander during meditation. When it happens, gently bring your focus back to your chosen point of attention, such as your breath.

Mindful Eating: Be mindful of what you eat by savoring each bite and paying attention to flavours, textures, and the act of nourishing your body.

Gratitude Practice: Incorporate gratitude into your mindfulness routine. By doing this, you reflect on things you are thankful for.

Silence and Solitude: Occasionally practice complete silence and solitude to deepen your mindfulness experience.

Seek Guidance: Consider joining a meditation group or seek guidance from a meditation teacher or therapist. I set aside time every day to write and meditate. Meditation gives me a sense of calm, peace and balance that benefit my emotional well-being and my overall health. It also helps me to have better focus and concentration. Meditation improves my memory

Be Compassionate: Show kindness and compassion to yourself, especially if you find it difficult to stay focused or if your mind is busy.

Measure Progress: Reflect on how mindfulness and meditation are affecting your mental well-being over time.

Remember that mindfulness and meditation are skills that develop with practice. The benefits often become apparent as you integrate them into your daily life. These practices can help reduce stress, improve emotional regulation, enhance focus, and promote an overall sense of well-being.

CHAPTER FOUR:
Emotional Intelligence and Emotional Health

Emotional Intelligence (EI)

Emotional intelligence refers to the ability to recognise, understand, manage, and use emotions effectively in various aspects of life. It encompasses several key components:

Self-awareness: The ability to recognise and understand your own emotions, including their causes and impact on your thoughts and behaviours.

Self-regulation: The capacity to manage and control your emotional reactions, including stress, anger, and anxiety. This involves impulse control and adaptability.

Social awareness: The skill of perceiving and understanding the emotions and needs of others. It includes empathy, which is the ability to put yourself in someone else's shoes.

Relationship management: The ability to use your emotional awareness and regulation skills to build and maintain healthy relationships. This involves effective communication, conflict resolution, and collaboration.

Developing emotional intelligence can lead to better interpersonal relationships, improved communication, and enhanced decision-making. It can also contribute to greater emotional well-being.

Emotional Health

Emotional health, often referred to as emotional well-being or mental health, is the state of one's emotional and psychological condition. It involves:

Emotional resilience: The ability to cope with life's challenges, setbacks, and stressors in a healthy way. Emotionally healthy individuals can bounce back from adversity.

Positive emotions: Experiencing a range of positive emotions such as joy, happiness, and contentment. Emotional health is not solely the absence of negative emotions but also the presence of positive ones.

Self-acceptance: This includes, having a positive self-image and self-esteem, as well as being comfor-table with one's emotions and flaws.

Emotional Balance: Maintaining a balance between various emotions and not being overwhelmed by negative emotions like anxiety or depression.

Effective Coping Strategies: Knowing how to manage stress, seek support when needed, and engage in self-care practices that promote emotional well-being.

Healthy Relationships: Building and maintaining healthy, supportive, and fulfilling relationships with others.

Emotional health is crucial for overall life satisfaction and functioning. It influences one's ability to handle stress, make decisions, and navigate life's challenges effectively.

Developing emotional intelligence can contribute to emotional health by providing the tools and skills needed to recognise, manage, and understand one's own emotions and the emotions of others. Cultivating both emotional intelligence and emotional health can lead to a more fulfilling and harmonious life.

Understanding Emotions and Their Impact on Overall Well-being

Understanding emotions and their impact on overall well-being is crucial for leading a healthy and fulfilling life. Emotions are complex, multi-faceted experiences that influence our thoughts, behaviours, and physical health. Here are some key points to consider:

Emotional Awareness: Recognising and labelling your emotions is the first step. It is important to be in touch with what you are feeling and why.

Emotional Intelligence: This involves not only understanding your own emotions but also being empathetic towards others' emotions. It can improve your relationships and communication skills.

Emotion Regulation: Learning how to manage and cope with different emotions can prevent them from negatively impacting your well-being. Techniques like mindfulness, deep breathing, and meditation can be helpful.

Positive Emotions: Cultivating positive emotions like gratitude, joy, and love can boost your overall well-being and resilience in the face of challenges.

Negative Emotions: It is also important to acknowledge and address negative emotions like anger, sadness, or fear. Suppressing them can have detrimental effects on mental and physical health.

Social Connection: Building and maintaining strong social connections can provide emotional support and enhance well-being. Humans are inherently social beings, and loneliness can negatively impact emotions and health.

Physical Health: Emotions can have a direct impact on physical health. Chronic stress, for example, can lead to a range of health problems. Managing stress and negative emotions is essential for maintaining overall well-being.

Seeking Help: If you find it challenging to manage your emotions or if they significantly affect your well-being, seeking the help of a therapist or counsellor can be beneficial. They can provide tools and strategies for emotional regulation and coping.

In summary, emotions play a vital role in our lives, and understanding and managing them can greatly influence our overall well-being. Developing emotional intelligence and adopting healthy strategies for dealing with emotions can lead to a happier and more fulfilling life.

Techniques for Managing and Expressing Emotions in a Healthy Way

Identify and Label Emotions: Start by recognising and labelling your emotions. This self-awareness is the first step in managing them effectively.

Mindfulness and Meditation: Practise mindfulness and meditation to stay present in the moment. This can help you observe your emotions without judgment and respond to them more consciously.

Deep Breathing: Take slow, deep breaths to calm your nervous system when you're feeling overwhelmed or anxious. This can help regulate your emotions.

Journaling: Keep a journal to express your thoughts and feelings. Writing can be a therapeutic way to process and understand your emotions.

Talk to Someone: Share your feelings with a trusted friend, family member, or therapist. Talking about your emotions can provide validation and support.

Physical Activity: Exercise releases endorphins, which can improve your mood and help you manage stress and anger.

Healthy Lifestyle: Prioritise sleep, nutrition, and hydration. These factors can significantly impact your emotional well-being.

Practise Empathy: Try to understand others' perspectives and feelings. This can lead to healthier communication and more harmonious relationships.

Set Boundaries: Establish clear boundaries in your personal and professional life to prevent emotional overwhelm.

Use Positive Self-Talk: Challenge negative thoughts with positive affirmations. Be kind and compas-sionate to yourself.

Seek Professional Help: If you are struggling to manage your emotions, consider seeking help from a therapist or counsellor. They can provide guidance and support tailored to your needs.

Creative Outlets: Engage in creative activities like art, music, or writing to channel and express your emotions in a constructive way.

Remember: Everyone's emotional journey is unique, and it is okay to seek help when needed. Finding the right combination of techniques that work for you may take time, so be patient with yourself as you navigate your emotions in a healthy way.

Building and nurturing meaningful relationships for emotional support

Communication: Open and honest communication is key to understanding each other's needs and feelings.

Empathy: Show empathy and actively listen to friends and loved ones to create a supportive environment.

Quality Time: Spend quality time together, whether in person or virtually, to strengthen your bonds. Do away with your mobile phones at times to minimise distractions.

Trust: Trust is the foundation of any meaningful relationship; be reliable and dependable.

Conflict Resolution: Learn to resolve conflicts constructively to maintain a healthy connection.

Give and Take: Relationships thrive on reciprocity; be willing to give support as well as receive it.

Boundaries: Set healthy boundaries to maintain your emotional well-being.

Diverse Connections: Build a network of relationships to ensure you have various sources of support.

Remember, nurturing these connections takes time and effort, but the emotional support gained is invaluable.

CHAPTER FIVE: Finding Purpose and Meaning

Finding purpose and meaning in life is a deeply personal and ongoing journey. It often involves self-reflection, exploration, and alignment with your values and passions. Some steps to consider:

Self-Reflection: Take time to think about what truly matters to you and what brings you joy and fulfillment.

Identify values: Clarify your core values and the principles that guide your decisions and actions.

Explore Your Passions: Discover activities or interests that resonate with you and make you feel engaged.

Set Goals: Establish meaningful goals that align with your values and passions, providing a sense of purpose.

Help Others: Acts of kindness and service can give a sense of purpose and meaning.

Learn and Grow: Continuous learning and personal development can lead to a more fulfilling life.

Connect with Others: Building meaningful relationships and a sense of community can enhance your sense of purpose.

Embrace Challenges: Overcoming obstacles and setbacks can lead to personal growth and a deeper sense of purpose.

Remember, finding purpose is a lifelong process, and it may evolve over time. Be patient with yourself and stay open to new experiences and insights.

Discovering Personal Values: Discovering your personal values is a meaningful journey. To align them with daily life, try these steps:

Self-Reflection: Take time to reflect on what truly matters to you. Consider your past experiences, what brings you joy, and what you are passionate about. It is always good to have a passion for something before you venture into the task.

Identify Core Values: List the values that resonate with you the most, such as honesty, creativity, or compassion.

Prioritise Values: Rank your values in order of importance. This helps to clarify what matters most when making decisions.

Evaluate Current Life: Assess how well your daily life aligns with your identified values. Are there areas where there is a disconnect?

Make Adjustments: Adjust your daily routines, decisions, and goals to better reflect your values. This might involve setting new priorities or making changes in your career, relationships, or hobbies.

Seek Support: Share your values with friends or a therapist for feedback and accountability.

Remember, aligning your values with daily life is an ongoing process, and it is okay to make gradual changes over time.

Exploring passions, Interests, and Talents to Create a Fulfilling Purpose

Exploring your passions, interests, and talents is a great way to discover your purpose. Start by reflecting on what activities or topics genuinely excite you. Consider how you can use your talents and interests to make a positive impact on the world or help others. Experiment, learn, and don't be afraid to adapt your path as you discover more about yourself. It is a lifelong journey towards finding fulfillment and purpose.

Setting Goals and Defining Success Based on Individual Aspirations

Setting goals and defining success based on individual aspirations is a highly personalized and empowering process. It involves:

Self-Reflection: Take time to understand your values, passions, and long-term desires. Consider what truly matters to you in life.

SMART Goals: Create Specific, Measurable, Achievable, Relevant, and Time-bound (SMART) goals that align with your aspirations. This helps make your goals concrete and actionable.

Prioritisation: Rank your goals by importance and feasibility. Focus on the ones that resonate most with your aspirations.

Visualise Success: Imagine what success looks like for each goal. This mental imagery can motivate and guide your actions.

Break It Down: Divide larger goals into smaller, manageable steps. This makes progress more achievable and less overwhelming.

Adaptability: Be open to adjusting your goals as circumstances change or as you gain new insights about your aspirations.

Measure Progress: Regularly evaluate your progress and make necessary adjustments to stay on track.

Celebrate Milestones: Acknowledge and celebrate your achievements along the way, no matter how small. It can boost motivation.

Learn from Setbacks: Do not be discouraged by setbacks; instead, see them as opportunities to learn and grow.

Personal Definition of Success: Define success on your terms, not based on others' expectations. It should reflect your values and aspirations, not societal pressures.

Remember that success is a dynamic and evolving concept. It's essential to adapt your goals and definition of success as you grow and change as an individual.

Strategies for Staying Motivated, Resilient, and Adapting to Change

To stay motivated, resilient, and adapting to change:

Set Clear Goals: Define specific, achievable goals to give yourself a sense of purpose and direction.

Stay Positive: Cultivate a positive mindset and focus on the benefits of change rather than dwelling on the challenges. I always look at the positive side of life.

Embrace Change: Accept that change is a natural part of life and an opportunity for growth. Change is the only constant thing in life.

Build Resilience: Develop resilience by learning from setbacks and developing coping mechanisms.

Seek Support: Lean on friends, family, or colleagues for emotional support and advice during times of change.

Stay Organised: Use tools like to-do-lists and calendars to stay organised and reduce feelings of overwhelm. To-do-lists, always help someone to be organised and carry out his daily activities very well.

Continuous Learning: Keep learning and acquiring new skills to adapt to evolving circumstances. Learning never ends. Engage in activities that stimulate your mind and promote personal growth.

Break Tasks into Smaller Steps: Divide big tasks into smaller, manageable steps to make progress feel less daunting.

Celebrate Achievements: Celebrate your successes, no matter how small, to boost motivation and confidence.

Self-Care: Prioritise self-care through activities like exercise, meditation, and adequate sleep to stay physically and mentally healthy.

Adaptability: Cultivate adaptability by being open to new ideas and flexible in your approach.

Visualise Success: Imagine yourself successfully navigating through change, which can help build confidence.

Time Management: Develop effective time management skills to make the most of your time and energy.

Stay Informed: Keep up with information that are relevant to the changes you are facing. This will help you to make informed decisions.

Take Breaks: Do not forget to take breaks and recharge when needed to avoid burnout.

Remember that everyone's journey is unique, and that it's okay to seek professional help if you're struggling to adapt to significant changes or facing mental health challenges during the process.

CHAPTER SIX: Balancing Work and Life

Balancing work and life is crucial for optimal well-being. Consider setting boundaries, prioritising self-care, and time management to achieve this balance.

Creating a Work-Life Balance that Promotes Well-Being

Creating a work-life balance that promotes well-being involves:

Setting Boundaries: Define clear boundaries between work and personal life. Stick to designated work hours and avoid bringing work-related tasks into your personal time.

Prioritising Self-Care: Make time for self-care activities like exercise, meditation, or hobbies to recharge and reduce stress.

Time Management: Efficiently manage your time at work by prioritising tasks and minimising distractions to prevent overworking.

Unpluging: Disconnect from digital devices and work emails during non-working hours to disconnect mentally from work.

Quality Family Time: Spend quality time with family and friends to nurture personal relationships.

Delegating and Asking for Help: Do not hesitate to delegate tasks at work and ask for help when needed to reduce overwhelm.

Vacation and PTO: Take regular vacations and use your paid time off to relax and rejuvenate.

Flexible Work Arrangements: Explore flexible work options like remote work or flexible hours, if possible.

Learn to Say No: Avoid overcommitting to work or social obligations. Saying no when necessary is crucial for balance.

Reflect and Adjust: Periodically assess your work-life balance and make adjustments as needed to maintain your well-being.

Achieving a healthy work-life balance is an ongoing process that may require trial and error to find what works best for you.

Effective Time Management Techniques and Strategies for Setting Boundaries

Effective time management techniques and strategies often involve setting clear boundaries to maximise productivity and maintain a healthy work-life balance.

Here are some key tips:

Prioritise Tasks: Identify your most important and time-sensitive tasks. Use techniques like the Eisenhower Matrix to categorise tasks into four quadrants: urgent and important, important but not urgent, urgent but not important, and neither urgent nor important.

Set SMART Goals: Make your goals Specific, Measurable, Achievable, Relevant, and Time-bound. These will help you to stay focused and motivated.

Create a to-do-list: List your daily tasks and organise them by priority. Tackle high-priority items first.

Time Blocking: Allocate specific blocks of time for different tasks or activities. This helps you concentrate on one thing at a time and prevents multitasking.

Learn to Say No: Do not overcommit yourself. Politely decline additional tasks or responsibilities that don't align with your goals or would overwhelm you. Some people like to commit themselves in activities they will not be able to carry out.

Limit Distractions: Identify common distractions, such as social media or constant email checking, and set boundaries to minimise them during work hours.

Delegate Tasks: If possible, delegate tasks that can be done by others. This frees up your time for more critical responsibilities.

Use Technology Wisely: Utilise productivity tools and apps to help manage your time and tasks efficiently.

Take Regular Breaks: Short breaks can improve focus and prevent burnout. Use techniques like the Pomodoro Technique (working for 25 minutes, then taking a 5-minute break) to maintain productivity.

Set Boundaries: Establish clear boundaries between work and personal life. Define specific work hours and stick to them to maintain a healthy work-life balance.

Practise Self-Care: Prioritise self-care activities like exercise, meditation, and proper sleep to recharge and stay productive.

Reflect and Adjust: Regularly assess your time management strategies and make necessary adjustments to improve your efficiency and well-being.

Remember that effective time management is a skill that takes practice and adaptation to your unique circumstances. Experiment with different techniques to find what works best for you and your specific goals.

Prioritising Self-care and Leisure Activities to Avoid Burnout

Prioritising self-care and leisure activities is essential to prevent burnout. Make time for activities that relax and rejuvenate you, such as hobbies, exercise, or simply unwinding. Setting boundaries and managing your workload can also help to maintain a healthy work-life balance.

Fostering Positive Relationships in the Workplace

To foster positive relationships in the workplace is crucial for a harmonious and productive environment. Here are some helpful tips:

- **Communication:** Open and honest communication is key. Encourage team members to express their ideas and concerns.

- **Respect:** Treat colleagues with respect and empathy. Valuing diversity and different perspectives is essential.

- **Collaboration:** Encourage teamwork and collaboration. Recognise and reward group achievements. In your office, give awards to deserving staff. It will boost their moral. It is also good to send your workers for training.

·   **Feedback:** Provide constructive feedback and be open to receiving it. This helps in personal and professional growth.

·   **Recognition:** Acknowledge and appreciate the efforts and contributions of your colleagues.

·   **Conflict Resolution:** Address conflicts promptly and professionally, focusing on finding solutions rather than blame.

·   **Work-Life Balance:** Promote a healthy work-life balance to prevent burnout and maintain well-being.

·   **Social Activities:** Organise team-building events or social activities to build camaraderie.

·   **Leadership:** Lead by example. Demonstrate positivity, fairness, and a commitment to the well-being of your team. Followers always like to emulate good leaders.

·   **Training:** Offer training in communication and interpersonal skills to enhance relationships.

CHAPTER SEVEN: Cultivating Positive Habits and Practices

Cultivating positive habits and practices can greatly enhance your well-being and productivity. Start by setting clear goals, creating a routine, and staying consistent.

· **Identify Your Goals:** Determine what positive changes you want to make in your life, whether it is improving your health, productivity, or relationships. I always perform self-evaluation for myself everyday. This self-evaluation makes me to discover the area of my life that I have improved.

· **Start Small:** Begin with manageable changes to avoid feeling overwhelmed. This will gradually build up to more significant adjustments.

· **Create a Routine**: Establish a daily or weekly schedule that incorporates your desired habits. Consistency is key to forming habits.

· **Use Reminders:** Set alarms, calendar events, or sticky notes to remind yourself to practise your chosen habits regularly.

· **Track Progress:** Keep a journal or use an app to monitor your progress. This can help you to stay motivated and see your improvement over time.

· **Accountability:** Share your goals with a friend or family member who can hold you accountable and provide support.

· **Be Patient:** Habits take time to develop. Don't get discouraged by setbacks; instead, learn from them and keep moving forward.

· **Stay Positive:** Maintain a positive attitude and focus on the benefits of your new habits. Also ensure to celebrate your successes along the way.

· **Self-Care:** Ensure you prioritise self-care to maintain the energy and motivation needed to sustain positive habits.

· **Adjust as Needed:** Be flexible and willing to adapt your habits and practices if they are not working as expected. Continuous improvement is key.

Understanding the Power of Habits and Their Impact on Well-Being

Habits play a significant role in well-being. They can influence our physical, mental, and emotional health. Positive habits like regular exercise, healthy eating, and mindfulness can improve overall well-being, while negative habit like smoking can harm it. Habits can shape our routines, mindset, and even our long-term health outcomes. Building and maintaining good habits can lead to a happier and healthier life.

Identifying Negative Habits and Replacing Them with Positive Ones

Identifying negative habits and replacing them with positive ones is a great way to improve your life. Here is a simple process to help you get started:

Self-Awareness: Begin by identifying the negative habits you want to change. This might involve behaviours like procrastination, overeating, smoking, or excessive screen time. Be honest with yourself about what needs to change.

Set Clear Goals: Define specific, achievable goals for the positive habits you want to establish. For example, if you want to exercise more, set a goal to work out for 30 minutes a day, five days a week.

Understand Triggers: Pay attention to situations or emotions that trigger your negative habits. This awareness will help you anticipate and address them effectively.

Replace, Do Not Eliminate: Instead of trying to eliminate a negative habit outright, focus on replacing it with a positive one. For instance, if you tend to snack when stressed, replace unhealthy snacks with healthier options like fruits or nuts.

Start Small: Begin with manageable changes. Trying to completely overhaul your life overnight can be overwhelming. Small, consistent steps are more sustainable.

Use Positive Reinforcement: Reward yourself for sticking to your positive habits. This can be as simple as acknowledging your progress or treating yourself when you reach milestones.

Be Patient: Changing habits takes time and effort. Expect setbacks along the way, but do not get discouraged. Stay committed to your goals and keep moving forward.

Remember that the key to success is persistence and consistency. Over time, these positive habits can become ingrained in your daily life, leading to lasting improvements in your well-being.

Incorporating Gratitude, Self-Reflection, and Personal Growth Practices

Incorporating gratitude, self-reflection, and personal growth practices into your daily routine can have a profound impact on your well-being and personal development. Here are some tips for incorporating these practices:

Gratitude: Start or end your day by jotting down a few things you're grateful for. It could be as simple as a good cup of coffee or a supportive friend.

Self-Reflection: Dedicate time to self-reflection regularly. Ask yourself questions about your goals, values, and experiences. Journalling can be a powerful tool for this.

Mindfulness Meditation: Incorporate mindfulness or meditation exercises into your routine. These practices can help you become more self-aware and reduce stress.

Reading and Learning: Make a habit of reading books or articles that inspire personal growth. Continual learning is a key component of personal development.

Goal Setting: Set clear and achievable goals for yourself. Regularly review your progress and adjust your goals as needed.

Surround Yourself Positively: Spend time with people who support and uplift you. Positive relationships can be a catalyst for personal growth.

Gratitude Journal: Consider keeping a gratitude journal where you write down things you're grateful for daily. This reinforces a positive outlook.

Practise Patience: Personal growth takes time. Be patient with yourself and recognise that setbacks are a natural part of the process.

Remember that personal growth is a lifelong journey, and it's okay to take small steps toward improvement. Consistency and self-compassion are key to making these practices a meaningful part of your life.

CHAPTER EIGHT: Environmental Well-Being

Environmental well-being refers to the state of harmony and balance between individuals and their surroundings. It encompasses how the physical environment, including nature and the built environment, affects our overall well-being. Here are some key aspects of environmental well-being:

Natural Environment: A healthy natural environment, including clean air, water, and green spaces, contributes to physical and mental well-being. Access to nature can reduce stress and promote relaxation.

Sustainable Living: Engaging in eco-friendly practices, such as reducing waste, conserving energy, and using sustainable resources, supports both personal and environmental well-being.

Outdoor Activities: Spending time outdoors and participating in outdoor activities like hiking, biking, or gardening can improve physical health and emotional well-being.

Community Engagement: Being part of a community that values and cares for the environment can foster a sense of belonging and purpose.

Environmental Stewardship: Taking an active role in protecting and preserving the environment through actions like volunteering for conservation efforts or supporting environmental causes can enhance a sense of fulfillment and connectedness.

Sustainable Consumption: Making informed choices as consumers, such as purchasing eco-friendly products and reducing waste, can contribute to a sense of responsibility and well-being.

Reducing Environmental Stressors: Addressing environmental stressors like pollution or noise can lead to improved mental and physical health.

Connection to Place: Feeling connected to and appreciating the natural and cultural elements of your surroundings can enhance a sense of identity and well-being.

Education and Awareness: Increasing your knowledge about environmental issues and solutions can empower you to make positive choices for both your own well-being and the planet's health.

Advocacy: Engaging in advocacy and supporting policies that protect the environment can give individuals a sense of purpose and impact.

Overall, environmental well-being is inter-connected with other dimensions of well-being, such as physical, mental, and social well-being. Caring for the environment not only benefits the planet but also contributes to a balanced and fulfilling life for individuals and communities.

Recognising the Influence of the Physical Environment on Well-Being

The physical environment plays a significant role in influencing well-being. Factors such as air quality, green spaces, access to nature, noise levels, and the design of buildings can all impact our physical and mental health. For example, living in areas with clean air and easy access to parks or natural settings is associated with improved well-being. I have zero-tolerance for dirtyness. I try as much as possible to live in clean and decent environment. Conversely, exposure to environmental pollutants or high levels of noise can have negative effects on health. Additionally, the design of urban spaces and buildings can affect social interactions and community well-being. Recognising and addressing these environmental factors is essential for promoting overall well-being and quality of life.

Creating a Harmonious and Nurturing Living Space

Creating a harmonious and nurturing living space involves several key elements:

Declutter: Start by getting rid of items you no longer need or love. A clutter-free environment can promote a sense of calm and order.

Natural Elements: Incorporate natural elements like plants, wood, and stone to bring the outdoors in. This can create a soothing and balanced atmosphere.

Colour Scheme: Choose a colour scheme that resonates with you and promotes the mood you desire. Soft, neutral colours can create a sense of tranquility, while brighter colours can energise a space.

Lighting: Use a combination of natural and artificial lighting to set the right ambiance. Natural light can boost mood, while adjustable lighting can create different atmospheres throughout the day.

Comfortable Furniture: Invest in comfortable and functional furniture that suits your lifestyle. Arranging furniture to facilitate conversation and movement can make the space feel more inviting.

Personal Touches: Add personal touches like artwork, photographs, or meaningful decor items that reflect your personality and values. These can make your space feel unique and nurturing.

Organisation: Use storage solutions to keep things organised and accessible. This reduces visual clutter and makes it easier to maintain a harmo-nious environment. It makes the environment neat and clean.

Textures: Incorporate a variety of textures through textiles like rugs, curtains, and cushions. This adds depth and tactile comfort to the space.

Sensory Elements: Consider scents and sounds. Aromatherapy, soothing music, or soundscapes can enhance the ambiance and promote relaxation.

Balance: Pay attention to the balance of elements in your space. Ensure there's a balance between open and closed spaces, soft and hard surfaces, and minimalism and decoration.

Remember that creating a harmonious living space is a personal journey, and it's essential to prioritise elements that resonate with your unique preferences and needs. Regularly assess and adjust your space to maintain its nurturing qualities.

Physical Exercise: Outdoor activities encourage physical activity. Whether it is hiking, biking, or simply taking a walk in the park, these activities promote cardiovascular health, improve fitness, and help maintain a healthy weight.

The Importance of Nature and Outdoor Activities for Mental and Physical Health

Nature and outdoor activities play a vital role in promoting both mental and physical health. Here is why:

Stress Reduction: Spending time in nature helps to reduce stress levels. The natural environment offers tranquility and an escape from the demands of everyday life, which can lower cortisol levels and improve overall well-being.

Vitamin D: Sunlight exposure during outdoor activities helps the body to produce vitamin D, which is essential for strong bones, a healthy immune system, and overall health.

Mood Enhancement: Nature and outdoor settings have been linked to improved mood and reduced symptoms of depression and anxiety. The beauty of natural landscapes can have a calming and uplifting effect.

Creativity and Cognitive Benefits: Time in nature can enhance creativity and cognitive function. It allows for mental rejuvenation and a break from the constant stimulation of screens and urban life.

Social Connection: Outdoor activities often involve social interaction, fostering a sense of community and social well-being. Connecting with others in natural settings can improve relationships and mental health.

Mindfulness and Presence: Being in nature encourages mindfulness and being present in the moment. This mindfulness practice can reduce rumination and improve mental clarity.

Biophilia: Humans have an innate connection to nature, known as biophilia. Being in natural environments satisfies this intrinsic need and can lead to a greater sense of fulfillment and happiness.

Incorporating outdoor activities and spending time in nature as part of one's lifestyle can have profound and lasting benefits for mental and physical health. It is a holistic approach that contributes to overall well-being.

Minimising Exposure to Toxins and Creating a Healthy Living Environment

Minimising exposure to toxins and creating a healthy living environment involves several steps:

Indoor Air Quality: Ensure good ventilation in your home. Use air purifiers and consider adding indoor plants known for air purification, such as snake plants and spider plants.

Non-Toxic Cleaning Products: Use eco-friendly and non-toxic cleaning products to reduce exposure to harmful chemicals.

Natural Materials: Choose furniture and building materials made from natural, low-VOC (volatile organic compounds) materials, to reduce off-gassing.

Filter Tap Water: Invest in a water filter to ensure your tap water is free from contaminants.

Reduce Plastics: Minimise the use of plastic products, especially those with BPA and phthalates, which can leach into food and water.

Healthy Diet: Eat organic and locally sourced foods to reduce exposure to pesticides and other chemicals.

Reduce Electromagnetic Exposure: Limit exposure to electromagnetic fields (EMFs) by turning off electronic devices at night and keeping them away from your sleeping area.

Radon Testing: Test your home for radon, a naturally occurring radioactive gas that can seep into buildings.

Natural Pest Control: Use natural methods for pest control instead of chemical pesticides.

Reduce Stress: Stress can impact your health. Incorporate stress-reducing activities like medita-tion or yoga into your routine.

Regular Cleaning: Keep your living space clean and free from dust and allergens.

Proper Storage: Store food and chemicals properly to prevent contamination.

Awareness: Stay informed about potential toxins in products and make informed choices.

Remember that creating a healthy living environment is an ongoing process that requires vigilance and a commitment to making sustainable, toxin-free choices.

CHAPTER NINE: Overcoming Challenges and Resilience

Overcoming challenges often requires resilience, which is the ability to bounce back from adversity and keep moving forward. Resilience can be developed through various means, including:

Positive Mindset: Cultivating a positive attitude can help you reframe challenges as opportunities for growth.

Adaptability: Being flexible and willing to adjust your approach when faced with obstacles can make overcoming challenges easier.

Social Support: Lean on friends, family, or a support network for emotional support and advice during tough times.

Problem-Solving Skills: Developing effective problem-solving skills can help you tackle challenges more effectively.

Self-Care: Prioritise self-care practices such as exercise, meditation, and adequate sleep to boost your mental and emotional resilience.

Learn from Failure: See failures as learning experiences and opportunities for improvement.

Goal Setting: Setting achievable goals can give you a sense of purpose and direction, even in challenging times.

Seeking Professional Help: In some cases, seeking guidance from a therapist or counsellor can be beneficial when facing particularly difficult challenges.

Remember that resilience is a skill that can be developed and strengthened over time. This will help you to navigate life's ups and downs more effectively.

Strategies for Overcoming Obstacles and Setbacks on the Path to Well-Being

Overcoming obstacles and setbacks on the path to well-being requires a combination of resilience, self-care, and positive strategies. Here are some strategies to help you navigate these challenges:

Mindfulness and Self-Awareness: Practise mindfulness to become more aware of your thoughts, emotions, and reactions. This self-awareness can help you identify and address obstacles more effectively.

Set Realistic Goals: Break down your well-being goals into smaller, achievable steps. This can make it easier to track your progress and stay motivated.

Adaptability: Be flexible and willing to adjust your plans when faced with setbacks. Life is unpredict-able, and adaptability can help you maintain your well-being.

Self-Care Routine: Establish a consistent self-care routine that includes activities like exercise, meditation, and adequate sleep. These practices can boost your physical and mental resilience.

Positive Self-Talk: Challenge negative self-talk and replace it with positive affirmations. This can improve your self-esteem and help you to stay motivated during difficult times.

Learn from Setbacks: View setbacks as opportunities for growth. Analyze what went wrong, what you can learn from the experience, and how you can do better next time.

Time Management: Organise your time effectively to prioritise well-being activities. Balancing work, personal life, and self-care is essential for overall well-being.

Cultivate Resilience: Develop resilience by building coping skills and learning to bounce back from adversity. Resilience is a key factor in over-coming obstacles.

Practice Gratitude: Regularly reflect on the things you're grateful for. This can shift your focus away from setbacks and help you to maintain a positive outlook.

Connect with a Supportive Community: Join groups or communities that share your well-being goals. Connecting with like-minded individuals can provide motivation and a sense of belonging.

Remember that setbacks are a natural part of any journey toward well-being. By implementing these strategies and staying persistent, you can overcome obstacles and continue on your path to a healthier and happier life.

Building Resilience and Bouncing Back from Adversity

Building resilience and bouncing back from adversity is a valuable skill that can help you navigate life's challenges. Here are some strategies to help you strengthen your resilience:

Positive Mindset: Cultivate a positive outlook on life. Focus on opportunities for growth and learning in every situation, even during adversity.

Problem-Solving Skills: Develop effective problem-solving skills. Break down complex problems into smaller, manageable tasks, and work through them systematically.

Adaptability: Embrace change and be flexible in your approach to challenges. Recognise that life is constantly evolving, and adaptability is a key aspect of resilience.

Set Realistic Goals: Set achievable goals and celebrate your progress along the way. This can provide a sense of accomplishment and motivation.

Mindfulness and Relaxation: Practise mindfulness and relaxation techniques like meditation and deep breathing. These practices can help reduce stress and increase emotional resilience.

Learn from Adversity: View adversity as an opportunity to learn and grow. Reflect on what you have learned from past challenges and how it can help you in the future.

Maintain a Supportive Routine: Stick to a daily routine that provides structure and stability, even during difficult times. This can create a sense of normalcy.

Positive Self-Talk: Challenge negative self-talk and replace it with positive affirmations. Building self-esteem can enhance your resilience.

Build Resilience Muscles: Start with smaller challenges and gradually tackle larger ones. Each successful experience in overcoming adversity can build your resilience *"muscles"*.

Maintain Perspective: Keep perspective during tough times. Remind yourself that setbacks are temporary, and you have the ability to overcome them.

Learn Stress Management: Develop effective stress management techniques, such as time management, setting boundaries, and practicing relaxation exercises.

Remember that resilience is a skill that can be developed and strengthened over time. It is normal to face adversity, but with resilience-building strategies, you can bounce back stronger and more capable of handling life's challenges.

Seeking Support and Utilising Resources for Mental Health and Personal Growth

Seeking support and utilising resources for mental health and personal growth is essential for overall well-being. Here are steps you can take to access the help and resources you may need:

Reach out to Friends and Family: Start by talking to trusted friends and family members about your mental health and personal growth goals. They can offer emotional support and may have valuable insights.

Online Resources: Explore reputable online resources and self-help materials related to mental health and personal growth. There are many websites, articles, and books available that offer valuable insights and strategies.

Support Groups: Join support groups or communities that focus on your specific challenges or goals. These groups can provide a sense of belonging and a platform to share experiences and advice.

Mental Health Apps: There are numerous mental health apps available that offer tools for managing stress, anxiety, and other mental health concerns. These apps can be a convenient way to access support and resources.

Workplace Assistance: Check if your workplace offers employee assistant programmes (EAPs) or mental health services. Many employers provide resources to help employees cope with stress and personal challenges.

Educational Programmes: Consider enrolling in courses or workshops related to personal growth and well-being. Many organisations and online platforms offer these programmes.

Hotlines and Crisis Services: In times of crisis or when you need immediate help, reach out to crisis hotlines or services. They are available 24/7 to provide support and guidance.

Medical Professionals: Consult with a healthcare provider, such as your primary care physician, if you believe there may be underlying medical factors contributing to your mental health concerns.

Financial Counselling: If financial stress is affecting your mental health, seek guidance from financial counsellors or advisors who can help you manage your finances effectively.

Self-Help Books: Explore self-help books written by experts in the field of personal development and mental health. These books often provide actionable strategies for personal growth.

Community Resources: Investigate local community resources, such as community centres, libraries, or non-profit organisations that offer workshops, support groups, or counselling services.

Online Forums: Participate in online forums or discussion boards where individuals share their experiences and advise on mental health and personal growth topics.

Remember that seeking support and utilising resources is a sign of strength, not weakness. Everyone faces challenges, and there are numerous resources available to help you on your journey toward better mental health and personal growth. Don't hesitate to reach out and take advantage of these resources when needed.

Cultivating a Positive Mindset and Embracing a Growth-Oriented Perspective

Cultivating a positive mindset and embracing a growth-oriented perspective can lead to personal and professional development. It involves focusing on opportunities for learning, resilience in the face of challenges, and maintaining an optimistic outlook on life. This mindset can foster self-improvement and open doors to new possibilities.

Conclusion

Reflecting on the Journey Towards Optimal Well-Being

Reflecting on the journey towards optimal well-being is a valuable practice. It involves assessing your physical, mental, and emotional health, as well as identifying areas for improvement. This self-awareness can lead to making positive changes in your lifestyle, habits, and priorities to enhance one's overall well-being and quality of life.

Celebrating Progress and Embracing the Ongoing Process

Celebrating progress and embracing the ongoing process are essential components of personal growth and achievement. Recognising and celebrating even small accomplishments can boost motivation and morale, while understanding that growth is a continuous journey helps to maintain a long-term perspective. It is about finding joy in the steps you have taken and the ones still ahead.

Encouragement to Continue Prioritising and Integrating Well-Being Practices in Every Day Life

Continuing to prioritise and integrate well-being practices into your every day life is a wonderful commitment to your long-term happiness and health. Remember that self-care is not selfish; it is essential. By dedicating time and effort to practices that nourish your body and mind, you will not only feel better in the present, but also set a strong foundation for a healthier and more fulfilling future. Keep up the good work!

References

David Viscott M.D. (2015). Emotional Resilience.

Debbie L. Stoewen (2017). Dimensions of Wellness: Change Your Habit, Change Your Life.

Deepak Chopra M.D. (1990). Perfect Health. The Complete Mind/body Guide.

Frank Lipman (2019). How to be Well. The 6 Keys to be Happy and Healthy Life.

Gretchen Rubin (2009). The Happiness Project.

About the Book

The comprehensive guide to obtaining holistic health and happiness in all aspects of life, "Embracing Optimal Well-Being" is your definitive path to accomplishing these desires. To assist you on your journey toward a life that is full of vitality and harmony, this revolutionary handbook relies together cutting-edge research, timeless wisdom, and practical solutions.

I have delved deeply into the interrelated realms of physical, mental, emotional, and spiritual well-being in this extended edition of the book. In this course, you will learn how to create resilience, enhance mindfulness, and foster positive connections that enrich your life through a combination of scientific insights and practical advice.

In this book, novel methods of nutrition, exercise, and stress management are discussed, and the reader is provided with tangible ways to improve their physical health. In addition to this, it explores the significance of mentally clear thinking, emotional intelligence, and spiritual fulfillment, and it provides strategies that can help you align your inner self with your external objectives.

The book "Embracing Optimal Well-Being" is more than just a guidebook; it is a companion on your journey toward holistic wellness. Providing you with motivational anecdotes, activities, and guided reflections, enables you to make changes to your lifestyle that are sustainable and that will benefit your health and happiness over the long run. This book will give you the tools and motivation you need to transform your life from the inside out, whether you are looking to increase your energy levels, become more effective at managing stress, or develop your spiritual practice.

About the Author

Olaitan Onakoya is a multi-talented professional with a diverse background spanning education, finance, and healthcare. He obtained his bachelor's degree in Economics from the prestigious Olabisi Onabanjo University in Ago-Iwoye, Ogun State, laying a solid foundation in analytical and quantitative skills.

Driven by a passion for imparting knowledge, Onakoya pursued a Post-Graduate Diploma in Education from the renowned University of Ibadan, equipping himself with the pedagogical tools to effectively disseminate information to others.

With over a decade of experience in the healthcare sector, Onakoya has established himself as a healthcare professional dedicated to promoting well-being and financial health. His expertise lies in guiding clients towards achieving financial freedom through sound financial management strategies, empowering them to make informed decisions and improve their overall quality of life.

Beyond his professional pursuits, Onakoya has showcased his literary prowess as an author, contributing to the literary landscape with thought-provoking works that resonate with readers from diverse backgrounds.

Onakoya's multidisciplinary background and wealth of experience position him as a valuable resource for individuals seeking guidance on financial matters, educational pursuits, and overall wellness. His commitment to continuous learning and his ability to bridge different domains make him a respected figure in his field.

Individuals seeking to connect with Onakoya can reach out to him through various channels, including **WhatsApp** at wa.me/2349061560679

Facebook (Onakoya Olaitan)

Email: oyeyemiolaitan@yahoo.com